FROM FEAR TO FAITH

A Caregiver's Journey

REFLECTIONS ON FINDING HOPE
IN THE MIDST OF DESPAIR
by
Joyce Marie Sheldon

LORIMER

PRESS

Davidson, North Carolina
2006

FIRST EDITION
Published by Lorimer Press, Davidson, NC

Printed in China

LIBRARY OF CONGRESS CONTROL NUMBER: 2006927080

ISBN 978-0-9704651-8-4

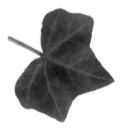

ACKNOWLEDGEMENTS

To those whose gifts of faith and courage have inspired me to be all that I can be —

My mother, Ruth, whose tender and graceful heart I admire;

My father, Frank, gone from this world for many years, but whose spirit guides me from afar;

Daniel Seufert, mountain wanderer and Irish dreamer, who inspired the writing of *The Three Steps*, *Glorious Dawn*, and *The Mountain Song*.

Leslie Rindoks, friend and woman tender of spirit and rich of soul.

And my husband, George.

> *We walked together on the journey*
> *— from fear to faith*
> *from tears to triumph —*

I love you all and will forever

For those lost in a sea of grief
may this book guide you
safely to shore.

CONTENTS

FAREWELL

TRIUMPH

PREFACE

WRITING has been a part of my life since childhood—from poems and essays in school, to romantic and spiritual prose in adulthood. When my husband was diagnosed with terminal liver disease in 1999, it was natural for me to express my thoughts and fears on paper. Writing was a release. Often I found myself at the computer in the early morning hours, pounding the keys in a desperate attempt to vent my frustrations, to let go of my grief, to soothe my spirit.

My husband spent two years traveling towards his death. We were determined it would be a journey of faith—not faith that he would recover miraculously, but faith that we could (and would!) accept the inevitable, trusting that God would provide strength and courage. We searched for something to give meaning to our days, a challenge to which we could direct our thoughts and energy. We would *live* our faith and teach our children, by example, how to die. We would provide a life lesson—or should I say a "death lesson." This would be our one last job to do together, the culmination of our life's work as parents.

My husband embraced this idea. He valued family above

all else and he worked hard to fulfill his part of the plan. Oh, yes, we struggled and faltered. But always, with the help of God, we picked ourselves back up and directed our hearts to the goal of living his last days and then, inevitably dying, in a manner worth remembering.

Since my husband died on January 12, 2001, my life has taken many twists and turns. Finally, I have settled near my children and grandchildren. I have wondered many times what value my poetry and prayers might have for others who find themselves walking the same road. Now, with the encouragement of friends and loved ones, I give this collection of prose, poetry and prayers to you. It is a record of my spiritual journey from fear to faith, from tears to triumph. It is an endless voyage, marked with sharp and jagged stumbling blocks and great rushes of sublime success. It is my hope that this book will aid and encourage you as you walk toward acceptance, peace and fulfillment.

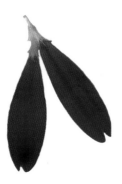

A Journey Begun

To become a caregiver is to lose oneself –
    to live in the silent shadow of disease or infirmity.

The focus of family and friends is on the person who is ill,
    as well it should be.

But meanwhile, the caregiver stumbles and falls,
only to have the cuts and scrapes go unnoticed and unattended.

Only one who has truly lived the silent role of caregiver
    can relate to the emotional highs and lows,
        the anger, the frustration, the guilt.

Caregiving is seldom a conscious choice.
It usually creeps up quietly, grabs one around the neck
and begins to squeeze – slowly and steadily.
The caregiver – tired and stressed –
becomes accustomed to the weight and pressure.
Only the slumping shoulders, the empty eyes,
tell the story of the heavy burden.

This is not to say caregiving is without miraculous graces,
rare opportunities for spiritual growth and sublime relationships.
    It is all these things!

In the end, however, it is the caregiver who survives
and who must learn to live again.
And I tell you now, you will never be the same!
This testimony of emotional and spiritual growth –
from fear to faith,
from tears to triumph –
records but a small portion of the emotions felt by the
unsung hero,
the caregiver.

It is in acknowledging this difficult task that you –
the caregiver –
are awarded your angel's wings.

DIS
BELIEF

Fig. 1

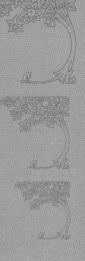

Fig. 3

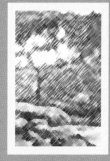

Fig. 2

OTHER PEOPLE

This is what happens
    to other people.

This is what happens
    on television.

    Six months –

How can this have anything to do
    with us?

Certain to hear news of a heart problem,
perhaps a necessary surgery.
A long and arduous recovery.
Rehab and
return to good health.

The doctor's face stern
His eyes sad, his lips tight.

Six months –
Six months –

No
hope?
No
magic drug?
No
history-making surgery?

Where is the script?
Quickly!
What do I say?

What do I *do?*
I do not know my lines.
The script – quickly, the script!

Is there a road map to show me
a safe route?
a short cut?

I watch. The color fades from his cheeks.

Tears well, but do not drop.
I will not let them.

Legs, weak.
I feel hot
and flushed
and cold
all at the same time.

Someone is talking to me –
    or is it ME talking to ME?
Are there questions?
Are there things to do?

What happens next?
What happens NOW?
The doctor's lips move.

A huge void fills my being
yet I am empty.
Darkness enters and crushes me into a million pieces.

Six months.
Six months.
Six months to live.

Me, Too

This is not about me.
This diagnosis is not about me.

　　　is it?

Joined in marriage,
　　　joined by 25 years together,
　　　joined by seven children.
Yes, this IS
　　　about me.
　　　We are one.

I have six months to live,
because without this man,
I will die also –

surely
definitely
positively.

There is no hope
for me.
I am dying, too.

Six months
begins

today.

One Last Job

It was a beautiful day. Even though my husband was in the hospital, I just *had* to be thankful for the fresh air and sunshine. Not a cloud in the sky!

But in my heart, a thunderstorm was brewing. Dark clouds, in the shape of a phone call from the clinic, gathered on the horizon. My husband had not met the qualifications for a transplant—our last hope for a miracle. Rain began to fall.

I sought assistance for the difficult job of telling my husband the disappointing news. His doctor was unavailable; the hospital chaplain had left. Even the nurses shunned my request for help. There was not a friendly face among them—no kind words, not a shoulder, not a soul to stand beside me.

And so, with a determined spirit, I proceeded to do it alone. My silent prayer was for strength and courage, and for the gift of saying the right words even though it seemed impossible that any words could be right in this situation.

Oh, it is amazing what gifts we receive just for calling out, and it would be proven to me that one is never, ever truly alone!

His room seemed exceptionally dark—like my spirit, dark and heavy with disappointment. My husband knew immediately that something was wrong.

"Please God," I said in my heart, "help me find the right words."

I told him the news. He was angry. He began to yell at the doctors who took the tests, the hospital, the system. I just stood there, praying.

And then God gave me the words.

"George," I said quietly, "Please listen." I took a deep breath. "There is one last job for us to do."

My husband waited for me to continue.

I cleared my throat and said, "There is one last job to do, and that is to show our children how to die with dignity and grace."

He looked at me in stunned silence.

In that moment we were exceedingly blessed!

He smiled. He took my hand. With the simple nod of his head, he agreed to the job at hand. We would, indeed, show our children how to die with dignity and grace.

For the next 24 months we worked together, accomplishing this one last job. We climbed mountains of joyous success and we fell into valleys of darkness and despair.

We had one last job to do and we were successful with the help of God.

One last job to do...

D/E SsPair

b

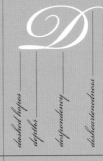

dashed hopes depths despondency disheartenedness

c

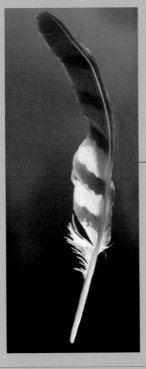

What is this
pounding in my
brain
That refuses to
rest
What is this
essence in my soul
That draws the
angels of
inspiration
To sit upon my
weary shoulders
Night after night

Denied

Free Me, Lord

I need to get away – I need to run away
from all the hopeless, helpless agony of my heart
to sit by silent streams
where no one sees my tears
or questions why no smile lights my face
I cannot breathe

The world no longer holds a single pleasure
The struggle seems no longer worth the effort
I cannot sleep
The silence of the night holds no repose for my soul
I cannot cry
The tears are buried under tons of grief

Do not call my name
No, not one more time, with needs I cannot meet
Is there someone I can talk to
who will listen to the emptiness of my heart
and fill it once again with long-lost joy
I pray it's You
Is it You, my God?

But I cannot hear your answer
I seek You everywhere
but cannot find the comfort or the peace
Where can I look?
I need You

I'm so tired, Lord
Don't You know that?
Am I selfish to want relief?
Why can't I sleep?
I did not know You would ask so much of me
and that I would be so weak
But look again, Lord
I'm dying, too
and I didn't know this would be your plan

I'm crying now
The tears are here
Will this be the relief?

Free me, Lord
Whatever it takes
I cannot understand the meaning
I am only human and cannot understand your plan
But, please, I pray, understand
and forgive your weak servant
I am so tired
I cannot sleep
Help me

12/00
3 a.m.

PURPOSE

My writing
has taken on a life of its own
I am unable to eat or sleep
until the words are finished
pouring from my restless heart
My fingers tap the cold keys
as if dancing
to a rhythm I cannot stop
The music and the tune
are not my own
but come to me from another place
O Lord, let the throbbing
of my heart be quieted.

I cannot sleep
and cannot stop
the relentless unloading
of my soul's despair
Or is it the despair
of all humanity
that I am doomed to bear?

It lies asleep
buried in the depths
of my tortured soul
only to be awakened
in these moments,
these hours,
when sleep should be my comfort
but is denied.

What is this pounding in my brain
that refuses to rest?
What is this essence in my soul
that draws the angels of inspiration?
They sit upon my weary shoulders
night after night.

01/15/06

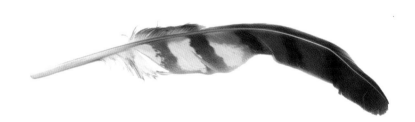

LOST

I am lost
on a sea of grief
The boat is being tossed
on treacherous waves
of despair.
Dark and lonely
I cannot see the shore –
There is no moonlight
to guide me.
I cannot imagine
the end of this voyage –
The thought
is too difficult
to bear.
There is no safe harbor,
no strong dock
with ropes
and lines
to secure this ship.
I beg
for the journey to end
and then
again,
beg
for it to continue.
Which is worse?
The road I walk
or the end
of the road?

Just One

Just one night
To sleep
To dream a peaceful dream
To awaken
Spirit rested
Soul refreshed

Just one morning
To walk among the angels of the earth
Head held high in courage
Unyielding to the pain
To dance the dance of the victorious
To fly as angels on the wing
To sing

Just one afternoon
To walk with the exalted
To hold the hand of those
Who share my plight
To touch the souls of kindred spirits
To share
To weep
To feel the understanding

Just one evening
To warm my spirit
Near radiant fires rich in goodness

To pray in quiet solitude
And joyful grace
To reach the heights
Of glorious repose

Just one night
To sleep
To dream a peaceful dream...

11/16/00
4 a.m.

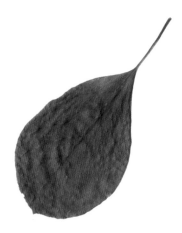

THE AUTUMN HEART

My heart has moved to autumn
The leaves of my soul
have gone from vibrant red and gold
to silent shades of brown

How soon they fell
from trees once great and tall
to crumble under footsteps
and become leaves no more

Soon winter comes –
the solitude,
the solitude

I hold tightly to the hope
that spring will once again engulf my spirit –
that life will be awakened in my soul

But I know – I know
only after the cold
and icy snow

6-19-00

No Glory

The day holds no glory
The dawn has no promise
The evening no solace
The night no repose
The heart has no freedom
The soul softly wanders
The mind lives in numbness
The end is so near

12/00

Imagine The Darkness Escaping
—A Meditation—

Sit quietly for a few minutes and clear your mind of the chaos of the day.

Feel your breath as you inhale and exhale.

Listen for the sound of your heart beating.

Concentrate on a blue abyss of nothingness.

Now,
Feel a relaxing sensation starting at the tip of your toes.
Feel this sensation as it moves into your feet and climbs into your legs.
Let go of the tension.
Relax.
You are totally at ease.
Picture a peaceful spirit entering your chest, your neck, your arms and fingers.
You are completely at peace with your body.

Now,
Imagine your heart – not a physical heart, but an imaginary heart.
Either something heart-shaped or a great white circle of light.
This is the sacred center of your precious being.
Embrace this heart as uniquely your own.
It belongs only to you.
It is sacred.
It is blessed.

Now,

Visualize as part of your heart all the dark areas of your past.
Imagine the hurts, the disappointments, the anger,
that are taking up precious space in your heart.
Be not fearful of their shadows.

Now,

Imagine an opening in the lower right-hand corner of your heart.
Through this hole all the darkness is pouring out.
The black and blue bruises of your life are escaping in a steady stream.
The darkness is escaping from your body—gone forever.
It has no place in your heart any longer.
Do not cling to it like an old friend,
but instead, release it with gratitude for the lessons learned.

Now,

Leave a small opening from which any future hurts can quickly escape.
Get rid of them as soon as they occur.

The good things in your heart are rejoicing now
because they have more room.
They are comfortable.
They can breathe and grow.
The good things in your heart are stretching and smiling.
Picture this! Feel the jubilation!
Imagine the joy in your heart because of the mass exodus of darkness.

Now,

Picture an opening in the upper left-hand corner of your heart.
Envision it surrounded by a great and brilliant light.
This light is silver and gold and it sparkles with goodness.

This is YOUR light, and yours alone. Your true and Godly light.
Through this light enter all the good things you have ever wanted and
needed —

> *Peace*
>> *Serenity*
>>> *Goodness*
>>>> *Patience*
>>>>> *Kindness*
>>>>>> *Understanding*
>>>>>>> *Forgiveness.*

As these good things enter, they are magnified a hundred fold by your
gentle spirit.

Your heart is comfortable.
It is peaceful.
It is clean and pure.
Your heart is healed of anger and disappointment.
Your heart is glowing with joy and serenity.

Now,
May you be blessed with the healing spirit of our Father
and may He bestow upon you a new sense of calm and self worth.

Now,
Rest in the spirit of the Lord.

Breathe
Relax
Grow

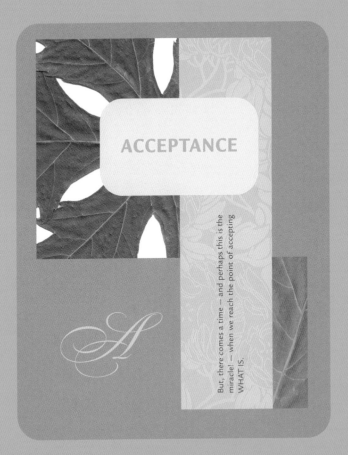

ACCEPTANCE

But, there comes a time — and perhaps this is the miracle! — when we reach the point of accepting WHAT IS.

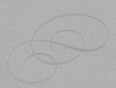

THREE STEPS

A friend asked what I learned from my husband's death. It took a few minutes to come up with an answer. Then, three words came to me: acceptance, serenity and respect.

It is normal to pray for a miracle when someone we love is dying, to beg for a reprieve from a diagnosis we never wanted to hear. That's all right. But, there comes a time—and perhaps this is the miracle—when we reach the point of accepting WHAT IS.

WHAT IS is a diagnosis of pending death. Accepting this is not a sign of weakness. It is not a sign of giving up the good fight. Accepting WHAT IS is the first step toward maintaining the control that is left in our lives and the lives of our loved ones.

Accepting all the trials and tribulations that accompany terminal illness can free our spirits and allow us to proceed to the second step: serenity. There, we find peace of mind and peace of heart. With serenity of spirit we can create around us an atmosphere of calm and harmony where everyone involved is gently moved along to the third step: respect. In the end, it is possible to find respect for life and respect for death.

There is a way to welcome death as part of the natural progression of life, another step on the path that each of us will one day travel. Yes, perhaps by our standards it is too soon; the patient is too young; we will miss him or her too much. But, those feelings are about us, the living. If we think instead of the one who is dying, if we can respect the days and hours of life that remain, the journey becomes far less difficult.

Accept each day as a gift. Visualize each trial as the petal of a beautiful rose, and picture all your tears as dewdrops. Soon you will see the entire flower in all its glory. The sun will shine again. Your tears will evaporate. You will have experienced the awesome joy of helping one precious soul travel to eternity.

MERELY PLAYERS

Merely players are they
who walk across
the pages of my life –
adding or detracting
from the full story.

The chapters fly
and it's up to me to say
"I bless you for your gifts," or
"Lo, I'm sorry that I met you!"

As the book is closed
to gather dust upon the shelf of life,
may all the pages
filled with sunshine
and with sorrow
melt together in a saga
rich in goodness
and with sweet intentions.

May the theme
dwell for generations.
I loved you all
each page –
each chapter –
to the end.

3/21/01

Lord, I Hope This Day Is Good

It is amazing how comforting a morning ritual can become. The joy of hearing a favorite song, lighting a special candle or straightening bed linens can become sacred acts.

My husband lived his last weeks in a little house in the North Carolina mountains. Each morning as the sun rose, I would open the drapes with the silent prayer, "Lord, I hope this day is good."

I lit our welcome candle, a candle which spoke to the Lord that we welcomed His presence and feared not the journey toward death. The flame burned brightly throughout our day. During the evening hours, its sweet aroma filled the silence of the sickroom with comfort and peace.

Each morning I gazed out the bedroom window and saw cows grazing in the nearby fields, a stray cat hoping for breakfast, the fog burning off the mountain top. These events occurred like clockwork, just like the needs of my loved one.

My morning ritual included a prayer of hope—hope that I would make it through just one more day. That was all—just *one more day*. My prayer was for patience, for strength and understanding, for serenity and faith. And each day, as if by the greatest miracle, the prayer was answered.

My ritual included writing—that magical healing tool of putting words on paper—expressing the emotions which swelled up in my heart and mind and overflowed into tears. Writing was my release, my medication, my therapy.

I filled countless pages, pleading for release from the heavy load. There were prayers asking for an acknowment that the road would not be traveled alone. There was thanksgiving to God for His infinite wisdom and patience with me, and there was a request for help. And always, always, each day began with the refrain, "Lord, I hope this day is good!"

Create your daily rituals of peace and serenity.

Light the candle.

Hear the music.

Lift your heart to a place far above the sickroom to the chambers of heaven.

11-07-05

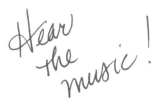

The Forever Friend

"This chair," I tell him, as I place it near his bed,
"is a place for your Forever Friend,
the One who will never leave you.

Reach to His hand for comfort,
when my hand is not enough.

Reach to His hand for understanding,
when human understanding cannot quiet your spirit.

He will be here always," I say.
"He will never leave you."

He likes the chair beside his bed
And in a feeble whisper often says,
"Move it closer, move it closer."

Indeed, the Forever Friend never leaves his side.
And when the welcome candle is lit and blessed,
and each morning – with the sunrise – is lit again,
the Forever Friend is always in the place
prepared for Him.

Nature runs its course – death and rebirth
outside the window,
it continues its endless cycle
in the sacred room –
the man in bed and his Forever Friend,
side by side – forever.

LISTEN!

LISTEN!
Your soul is longing for silence.

BELIEVE!
Faith dwells in the peaceful soul.

TRUST!
A child-like heart
moves forward in grace.

Meanwhile the body – worn and weak,
tried and tired –
unravels piece by piece.

Be silent

and listen.

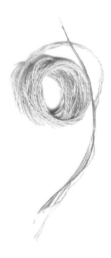

Carry Me

You carry me
across the sea of darkness

You shelter me
from wind and rain and cold

You strengthen me
with fortitude and courage

To fight these worldly battles
– dark, untold

Your hands reach out with comfort
– warm, tender

Your words resound
with peace and joy and love

Your Spirit gives me gifts
beyond all measure

You shower me with blessings

You are faith
    and hope
        and understanding

You carry me

Love and Trust

I feel like I am living someone else's life. I have stepped outside myself and now I observe another woman. This woman seems confident even under the worst of circumstances. I watch as she cares for her dying husband and am amazed at her ability to handle the exhausting tasks associated with his illness. She lifts him to the bedside commode and maintains dignity and grace for both of them. She bathes him with the richness of her love and combs his hair with the tenderness of a mother.

It is as though her very touch is magical. She heals his spirit because she knows she cannot heal his body.

I watch this woman share her faith and trust with the man who is dying. She writes poetry for him. She lights a welcome candle each morning and together they pray for acceptance, for a peaceful death and for the place in heaven reserved for those who suffer.

The love this woman exhibits begets more love and more love and the trust between the two of them begets more trust and more trust. The love and trust multiplies just like the loaves and the fishes in the Bible until the entire sick room is all about the *life* they share.

One day, as the sun rises over the mountaintop and burns away the morning fog, the woman speaks and her words echo in my ears:

"My Dearest,
The angels are coming to rescue you from the depths of your pain. The best and the highest are coming. The rose

and the silver, the blue and the gold. The angels are coming to carry your precious soul up out of your agony —to give you peace and serenity. *The angels are coming to rescue you.*

The man smiles and says,

"Dearest Love,
We have walked together down the road of life and you have shown me love and trust in good times and in bad. We have found peace and happiness like the missing pieces of a puzzle. Thank you."

The spirit of the woman I was joins with the woman I have become.

I vow to carry on

7/7/05
28*th* *wedding anniversary*

No Return

You've taken me upon a sacred voyage
from which I fear there is no safe return.
You've let my spirit soar beyond the heavens.
You've dragged my soul through agony and sin.

You've drowned my heart in waves of purple anguish
then saved me with your kind and gentle grace.
You've walked with me through tall and stately forests
and in the shadow let me see your face.

In tears and pain, You've been my faithful partner –
You've saved me from the darkness of the night.
And when my garden flowers hung in dryness
You've been the saving water, and the light.

Now that the journey's end has left me aching
You still engulf my every thought and dream.
You and I will walk forever bonded
'til both can rest by cool and heavenly streams.

3/21/01
3 a.m.

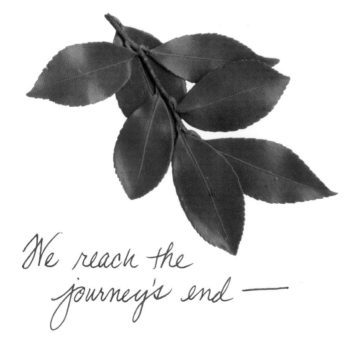

We reach the
journey's end —

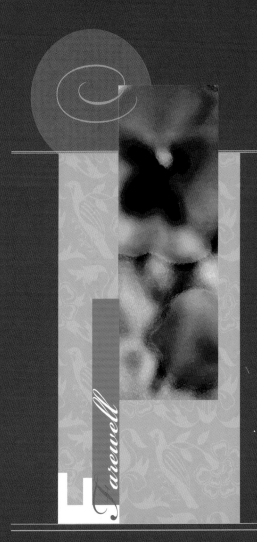

Farewell

...save me
from the
echo of his
voice within
my heart.

THE ANGELS ARE COMING

The angels are coming
to rescue you
from the depths of your pain.
The best and the brightest are coming –
the rose and the silver
the blue and the gold.
The angels are coming
to carry your precious soul
up – out of your agony –
to give you peace and serenity.
The angels are coming
to rescue you.

The angels are coming
to release you
from anxiety and fear.
They will leave behind
your withered body tortured with disease,
they will restore your gracious heart.
The angels are coming
to release you.

The angels are coming
to relieve you
of your human frailty.
They will bless you
with total contentment.
The angels are coming
to carry you
to the One Who loves you best,
to the One from Whom you first came,
The Lord, our beloved God,
and with Him
you will forever rest in peace.

The angels are coming ...
The angels are coming ...

7/00

THE OTHER WOMAN

One day, just before Thanksgiving, my husband informed me that he was in love with another woman—not what I wanted to hear when my days and nights for more than 18 months had been in devoted service to him. But then, with a little smile on his parched lips, he identified the "other woman." It was Reva, an older, southern lady of great compassion. An aide for Hospice, she visited every other day at first, then every day as the situation worsened.

Initially, my husband rejected Reva's offer to bathe him and wash his hair. He was a stubborn man and admitting that he needed help was yet another step on the road to acceptance. He eventually surrendered to Reva's gentle persistence.

Over the days and weeks that Reva tended to my husband's needs, and gave me a much-needed respite, he fell in love. Their eyes met on a level of stranger-to-stranger, then caregiver to patient, then friend to friend. They were both devoted to making the best out of what was happening.

He was dying and we knew it. Our prayer was for a peaceful death. Thanksgiving and Christmas loomed before us with more depth and meaning than ever. We knew these holidays would be our last together. As they approached, we asked for one more thing—to enjoy the season with our children.

Because of Reva, I could relinquish some of the caregiving. Because of Reva and her humility and kindness, I was sure my husband was being cared for with dignity and respect. Because of Reva, who on that last day took his blood pressure and looked at me with tears in her eyes, I was able to know, without words, that the end was near. And because of Reva, I was able to spend those last moments before the coma engulfed his spirit knowing the two of us—me and my husband's "new love"—had cared for this man in an exceptional way.

We had wonderful holidays that year. Although my husband was weak physically, he remained strong mentally. Like a king on his throne, he sat in a chair, surrounded by the family he loved so much. The joy on his face and the love in his eyes radiated throughout the room. Our seven children, their spouses, and our four grandchildren knew they were blessed to have this time together.

Our prayers were answered!

and joy radiates

Fear Revisited

He falls silent as another coma claims his body, his mind.
He ceases to move, to speak.
These quiet moments, these torturous hours,
linger like shadows against the morning wall
and fill my anguished spirit with fear.
Is this the last? I ask.
Will there be no return this time?
Has this ugly monster finally claimed all that was mine?

At first, I welcome the freedom of knowing
there will be no requests of me,
  no demands on my time,
  no questions that cannot be answered.
And then I am filled with longing for them all.
They give meaning to my existence.

Now I simply wait, patiently at first,
and then with tormenting unrest.
I sit
and watch
and wonder.

The old wicker rocking chair has been placed near the bedside
and I, the guardian of life,
  sit and rock
  and rock
   and rock.

Watching his chest rise and fall beneath the covers
becomes an obsession.
I stare at his mouth as if to force his feeble breath to continue.
My own heartbeat fills the room with sound
or is it just a frightening echo in my ears?

The horror of the dark night ahead panics my weakened soul.
The nightmare of the loss shakes my fading spirit.

I am alone.
I am afraid.
I weep.

A Love Story…

The room was quiet, the sun had set
and purple shadows cast a lovely glow
upon my loved one –
lying there –
mind and body weakened,
eyes fixed upon the ceiling.

He reached his feeble arm into the air –
up – and up some more –
as if to catch the hand of a beloved Friend.

Softly – oh, so softly, did he whisper,
"Take me home – take me home"
and even in his weakness
his head began to rise
up off the softness of the pillow
He gathered all his strength
and tried so hard to catch
the holy hand outstretched to him.
"Take me home," he said.

I wept with joy,
witnessing
this blessed moment when God arrived –
to take my humble loved one home

I pulled my shaky body
up from the floor where I had knelt

and grabbed my chest.
Sadness and joy swirled around together
in my aching heart.

"You can go," I said,
"reach out."
And then I left the two alone together.

Later, when I walked into that sacred space
he lay there peacefully, on his back
and said as clear as clear could be,

"I wanted to go, but I didn't see you there –
and so I didn't go.

I want to be with you."

"Turn me toward you," he said,
"and wrap me in your arms.

I want to be with you."

My shoulders shook and I wept
to know his love so true –
and I was glad to know that soon
he would find peace, at Home.

CONFESSION

I am weary.
My soul is shaken to its core.
My heart is heavy and in pain, and
you lie in a dreamless state while
I kneel at your side in constant prayer.
I pray that you be released from this prison;
pray that I can endure until the end.

If the face of death knocks at the door
would I open it?
Would I let you go?

I don't know.

I can't bear to watch you suffer.
My knees ache and sting.
I cannot rise to open the door.
I cannot leave your side.

For as long as breath is yours,
for as deep as you might sleep,
I will wait.
I am yours to keep.

THE PORCH

How many lonely nights will I sit on this porch watching the river as the moonlight casts its eerie shadows? I wonder how far the river flows. Could I possibly toss my cares into the dark waters and have them swiftly carried downstream? No, that would be too easy.

2 a.m. - 3 a.m. - 4 a.m.

I am still here—alone and afraid. Fear grips my heart and squeezes hard and long. I rub my chest to ease the pain.

Because I have deserted the bedroom for the serenity of the porch, the dying man lies alone, a coma for his companion, a candle for his comfort, music for his fading spirit.

I count the stars and notice one—just one—extra bright. It fascinates me. Is it winking? At me? "Could it be you, Daddy?" I ask out loud. Only the moon hears me.

Although he is gone from this world, calling out to my father has become a routine, a comfort. He has become my friend on this journey toward death. Tears stream down my face. "Can you help us?" I ask with the voice of a child.

My gaze moves slowly across the shadows of the dimly lit porch. I see the wilting flowers, once bright with life, once delicate in their texture; unfinished books with words of inspiration on their pages, just waiting to be opened once again; the wooden swing, silent and empty, its once colorful cushions now faded and cold.

I cannot throw away the flowers. That would be admitting that death lives here. I cannot finish reading the books. Then I would have come to the end. I cannot replace the cushions. New cushions will never know the essence of our beings.

The dying man in bed is the flower. Once bright with life, now wilting. I cannot give him up. Our life together lives in the unfinished books and I am afraid to read the last chapter. And the cushions on the swing—husband and wife—the fabric is dull, but the life is still precious.

Gazing back to the river, I feel a presence nearby, a soft touch on my shoulder. "Is it You, God?" I ask. "Are You here to take the books and the flowers and the old cushions? Is it time for us to give up our attachment to the things of this world?"

A soft breeze moves quietly through the trees and I hear the rustling of the leaves. The river glows as if someone has thrown stardust across it from shore to shore. The pages of an open book are blown from right to left as if being read swiftly, until the last page is reached. I fear the meaning.

My hand reaches out for the wilting flowers and I clutch them to my breast. I grab the book and keep it opened to the last page. I tremble as the old swing moves to and fro in the evening breeze.

"Don't take these from me," I beg. A voice speaks in the silence of my heart and a sense of peace and serenity fills my soul. There is a sense of joy in my heart. I am comforted.

"I must go to him," I say. But I cannot rise from the chair. The presence moves from the porch to the bedroom. I realize my place is here with the stars and the moon and not with the dying man and his guest. My place is here on the porch.

Through the window I see the candlelight flicker and die. The music fades, until I can hear it no more.

And the loving presence—the tender voice—brings peace and comfort and joy to my loved one. Together they leave me, hand in hand, and I am alone on the porch. A gentle rain begins to fall. I hear it as it lands softly on the spring grass. It dances on the river like little bubbles of happiness.

This is the last of life, the end for which we were born. Farewell, my husband, my friend.

My grip on the wilting flowers loosens. I gently close the book which is now finished. The swing is still. My task is done.

And I say out loud as I rest in solitude on the porch ...

> In my loneliness, I see your face
> I feel your spirit, drenched with grace
> I hear the flutter of angels' wings
> The sound of trumpets
> Echoing
>
> Till we meet again ...

7/11/05

TODAY IT ENDS – JANUARY 12, 2001

Today it ends
I know it in my heart
Death is at the door
He is dying
And I shall let him go
There is no fear –
Fear left this house
And in its place
Grace
Has been our companion
Our gift from God
Strength and courage
Have sheltered us from dread
Joy and thanksgiving
Have protected us from doubt

I wipe the frothy foam
From his parched lips
Evidence of the failing lungs
This is to be the last act of love
The last touch
of his breathing spirit

He will die today
I know it in my heart
I want to see his spirit soar
To the heavens

I want to watch his leaving
But God in His wisdom
Puts me to sleep by his side
And takes his precious soul
Home at last
I shall not witness his leaving
But I feel it just the same
My heart crashes
and lies empty on the floor
My spirit soars to the heavens

I tremble
at the glory
of it all

AFTER

Someone gently
takes me by the hand
and leads me
to the dimly lit room.
She helps me to the bed
fresh with crisp linens
pillows fluffed,
blanket warmed,
she guides me to its comfort
this cold and lonely morn.
Tenderly,
she wipes my tearful face
and like a child
gives a warm embrace.
I lie alone
and it seems strange –
no one to call my name –
I listen just the same.
I listen,
just the same.

And for 11 hours,
Yes, 11 hours I sleep.
Motionless,
No movement and no sound.

She watches
fearful I might follow him
knowing my soul is so filled with longing.
But, I remain with the living –
the breathing –
The people whom I love,
and who love me.
To her,
the devoted daughter.

But still,
I listen.

You Showed Me

You showed me strength
when I was weak
you gave me courage
to face the storms
and when the vicious waves
of life
tore apart
the boat we'd built
you threw a raft
to save me
together
we swam to the shore
you suffered quietly
in your chair
you watched and waited
while we grew
and when you were certain
we were strong
you made your move
and left us here
and we have
only one job to do –
to bless your memory
every day
to keep your name
in all our hearts
to live in peace
and joy and love
until we meet again

1/14/01

VALLEY OF PEACE

You live now in the Valley of Peace
With companions of Joy and Love and Mercy
Your life – a valiant voyage
Your heart – a courageous captain
Battles fought
Battles won
Battles lost
But in every step
A movement toward the end
Born of God
Died unto God
And in the end
Giver of gifts beyond your strength
To those in need of gifts
Courageous heart
Valiant spirit
You are never far from those you love

3/01

DEAREST ONE

Dearest One,

My heart is flooded with memories of you:
The last time I held your hand,
The last words you spoke to me.
Did you know you were leaving?
Why didn't you tell me?
I would have told you more often
that our life together was worth
the "bruised knees" and "broken bones."

You always apologized for the difficulties,
yet failed to realize
there is no road too hard to travel –
that two hearts bound in love
cannot walk along together.

Did you see heaven in those last hours?
I know you did!
There is no smile to compare
to the one upon your face that day.

My heart is flooded with memories.
My soul is heavy with the loss.
I cannot imagine life without you.
You have been my focus –
my every moment
was spent loving you.

Are you counting my tears?
When will they end?
My heart aches and I am lonely.
I long to see your face
just one more time,
to hold your hand and
hear you say you love me.

You were a treasured soul,
and perhaps it was only I
who understood your needs.

Your heart was frail,
your spirit longing
and in the end, it was only God
who could give you peace.

Do you see me now?
Please let me know.
I cannot see you
and my heart aches with the loss.

3/01

Dear Father

Dear Father,
We bless your holy name
and thank You for your presence in our lives.

Help us to move our hearts
from the valley of despair
to the mountaintop of faith.

Help us to accept your will
as divinely perfect and infinitely merciful.

Father, help us to release to You
the doubts and fears that plague our spirits
and to receive your blessing
of encouragement and acceptance.

Help us, Father,
to realize we are your beloved children
and that your grace
is always available to us
for the asking.

We detach ourselves
from the spirit of your son George,
whom You loaned to us
on this earthly plane,

and acknowledge that You alone
are our true Father.

Bless him, fill him with your love,
and take him safely to your holy dwelling place
that he might enjoy
eternal happiness.

Father,
we accept your holy will
and pray for the strength
to continue on our path to You,
to reach out to other family members,
and to remain centered on You.

Remind us there is good in all things
if we look beyond the obvious.

Take our suffering, Lord,
and make from it
a fragrant bouquet for your Blessed Mother.

Restore our faith,
and remind us You have never deserted us;
that it is we who have forgotten your presence
in every situation.

As You sit next to us now, Father,
we ask your blessing on our family.
Please touch our hearts,
keep us strong.
and bond us through adversity.

We ask this in the name of your Son,
Jesus Christ.

01/01/01
Dawn

THE SILENCE

The silence is deafening
bouncing off the cold plastered walls
of this small and lonely room,
leaving the echo of a haunting refrain.

Its dark shadows cast upon my aching heart
scars so thick and deep and red
left behind as a memory.

The silence is deafening.
My soul is dead.
He is gone now to another place –
a place I cannot see –
and though I know he lives in peace and joy,
what about me?

Oh, the silence is deafening.
He does not call my name.
He does not need my arms.
Sometimes, for a brief sacred moment,
I think I hear him call.
but he is gone,
after all.

Who Am I?

Who am I without you?

When you dreamed, I believed.
When you asked, I replied.
When you walked with tigers
I walked at your side.

When you were weak, my courage
enriched your aching heart.
What am I to do now
that we are apart?

Do I know who I am, dear,
without you at my side?
My world was you and you alone –

and then you died.

Now I walk alone here
on the plain of desert sand,
without you here to love me
and hold my lonely hand.

Can I give myself the courage
and the strength to carry on?
Can I speak and dream and walk the path
from dusk to early dawn?

All the gifts I gave away –
can I take them for myself?
Can I survive this cold ordeal
and cross the raging gulf

without you?

10/05

NOT THERE

Isn't it strange
how I think you are still there
sitting by the window,
waiting for my return?
I can almost see your face.

So I do not stop,
I do not linger anywhere.
I rush to see you
waiting.
But you're not there.

I sit alone.
My mind drifts
to thoughts of days gone by.
I feel a loving touch upon my knee
like a gentle breeze
whispering my name.
I sigh.
I call out your name
I open my eyes,
and you're not there.

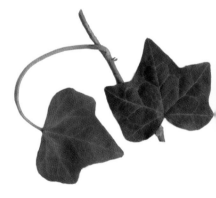

Every day that passes,
every night alone,
I move one step closer
to accepting you are gone.
But still,
I look for your face –
I wait for your touch.

But you're not there.

01/27/06

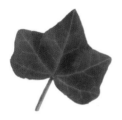

A Prayer

Deliver me, Lord, from the silence
which roams across my soul.
Like a gypsy across the arid plain
it smiles and it dances
to a rhythm I do not know.
I cannot catch my breath.
My feet are not moving to the beat.
Deliver me.

O Lord, save me from the echo
of his voice within my heart.
That painful, aching, plea for help
I tried so hard to fill.
It resonates with haunting tones,
I cannot bear the sound.
It hurts to hear the plaintive call.
Save me.

Cleanse me, Lord, from memories,
which cling like shadows in the night –
like wounds upon a soldier
like scars upon my heart.
They impair my vision
and cloud my every dream.
They dim the precious victory of the fight.
Cleanse me!

1/14/06

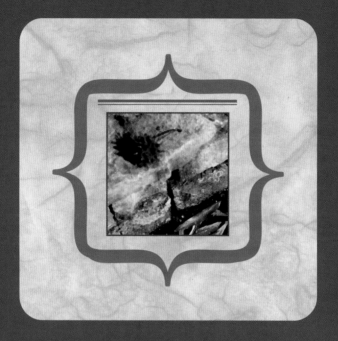

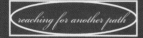
reaching for another path

GLORIOUS DAWN

Glorious dawn,
fog slowly lifting,
surprising me with majestic wonder.
My heart is bursting with joy
at the nearness of You.

You are my dearest love.
my constant companion.
You feed me goodness and light.
How is it that I forget You
at times along my journey?

You always wait
to be found once again,
my true love.

I beg You
wash the world
from my weary mind.
Cleanse my heavy heart
of things that have no meaning.
Fill me, I pray, with your gracious Spirit
that I might magnify it
to the world.

May your grace
be reflected in my eyes
to those who can truly see
and in my gentle touch
to those who can truly feel.

May my humble presence
be received joyfully
by those who search for You
and may my life be a tribute
to your precious
love and light.

5/01/05

my heart is bursting with joy!

WHEN I HAVE DIED...

When I have died
and all that you know of me
has ceased to be
weep not!
For I will be singing
and dancing
in the House of the Lord
and He will fill with awesome joy
that space in your heart
that misses me so much
and gently will He touch your cheek
and in that moment
all your tears will vanish

7/25/00

THE MOUNTAIN SONG

I sat among the glory of the clouds
on mountain top of grass and dew and sun
and felt the Hand of God upon my face
- this awesome Sunday morn

And in that bright and blessed moment,
that warm and loving, gentle Father's touch,
I realized the purpose of my living
- to love so much

To touch the sacred spirits of the living
to honor souls gone on to mansions gold
to bless your name and help you on your journey
- dear friend, with joy outpoured

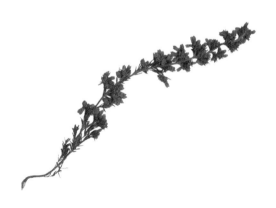

STEP OUTSIDE YOURSELF
—An Outdoor Meditation—

Take comfort in the glorious haven of nature. Sit outside by a brook or stream where you can hear the sound of water flowing.

Close your eyes. Rest your hands on your knees, palms upwards and be still.

Breathe.

Be mindful of the earth that surrounds you. Listen for the song of a single bird. Imagine its call as summoning you to the energy of the stream as it flows steadily and with purpose. This is the living water of the Higher Power.

Visualize this water as pure and glistening. Watch in your mind's eye as crystals of sunlight pour down out of the heavens and dance like little elves upon the ripples. Step outside your body and picture yourself reaching down to drink of this water. Scoop the water into your hands and satisfy your thirst for love and compassion. They will be yours and this vision will cleanse and fortify your spirit.

In your mind, picture the rocks over which the water travels. They are like life's stumbling blocks, but always, always, the water passes over them, reaching for another path to take. So, too, your troubles will travel over the rocks. Picture this. Your troubles are like droplets of water, crashing into the rocks and moving steadily toward a calm sea of peace and joy. Someday, this will all be behind you.

Imagine the trees, tall and stately, standing as pillars against the sky, soaring to the heavens. Smell the fragrance of the wood, the leaves, the blossoms. Use them as vehicles for your prayers. Move with the branches as they dance and sway in the breeze. Raise your arms in joy and thanksgiving.

This is the only moment!
This is the only breath to take!
This is the vision to which you must cling!
Listen closely to the silence. God is speaking to you. He will fortify your spirit. He will cleanse your soul. You have only to ask.

Sit
Breathe
Be mindful
Imagine
Ask
Listen

Receive !

5/01/05

AFTERWORD
—A Tribute to Hospice—

In 1998, my husband and I retired to Stuart, Florida. We bought a condo on the St. Lucie River and fulfilled his desire to have a pontoon boat. We dreamed of lazy days cruising down the river, enjoying the sun and relaxing. All dreams were cut short by the diagnosis of his terminal disease just three months later.

Eventually, we turned to the Hospice organization of Martin County for assistance. Their staff of nurses, aides, and social workers provided excellent care for my husband. In addition, they recommended I attend a caregiver's support group. This group of men and women met once a week, traveling together toward the unknown. Bound by common failures and victories, they shared the trials and tribulations associated with caregiving. For a long time, however, I rejected the offer of accepting help like this for myself. I believed that the focus should be entirely on my husband. Slowly, but surely, I realized that it was important to take care of myself, both physically and emotionally. Finding a way to not only understand my own feelings, but to share them with others, helped me become a stronger and more successful caregiver.

Attending my first caregiver's meeting, I couldn't even say my name for the tears. Someone quietly passed me a box of tissues. The next time was a bit easier. Eventually, I became an active participant in the discussions and found myself passing the tissues to the newest person in the group.

Towards the end of my husband's illness, we decided to live near our children so that they could visit more frequently and play a more supportive role in the caregiving. We moved to Waynesville, North Carolina, a small town in the Smoky Mountains. The strong, spiritual atmosphere there provided peace and serenity for my husband's last days.

Again, we contacted Hospice and they provided in-home assistance and guidance. They came with their expertise, their compassion, their friendship. From the nurse to the social worker, from the aide to the chaplain—each person brought gifts of beauty and joy and peace. Each person let us know we weren't alone on the journey. Being a step removed from family, they were able to approach situations from another perspective, without the emotions we were experiencing which sometimes clouded our decision-making.

In particular, I remember Dee Dee, George's nurse. She treated him with respect, but had a playful attitude and brought cheer to his days. She told him the hard truth and he accepted it from her. And Reva, a nurse's aide, who kept his body comfortable and his spirit comforted. How blessed we were to know them!

Now, five years later, I am a Hospice volunteer in Iredell County, North Carolina. Because I understand and sympathize with the role of caregiver, I direct my energies in that area, providing assistance and comfort to others who are saying good-bye to someone they love. It is one small way to say thank you to a wonderful organization called Hospice.

I don't know what we would have done without them.

MY CAREGIVER FRIEND

We walk along a road not of our choosing
and as we tread with honor and with grace…
Our heads held high, though hearts are strained,
we're nourished by the strength we give each other –
made strong by gifts of love and gifts of sharing
by moments filled with warmth and understanding
because we listen and we hear what each is saying…
The gentle touch upon a shoulder weary
A smile, a wink, a nod of sweet compassion so endearing.

You are my caregiver friend.
We are joined in spirit and in deed.
Please know my heart has been uplifted
and I pray for you every day –
You are my special friend,
my kindred heart upon the road unknown.
I am all the better for the knowing of your spirit.

We cannot depend upon our mere humanity
to make it through the darkest of our days.
We must rise above the simple body where we dwell
and as we rise, join – one soul unto the other –
to daily administer His love.

10/16/00
4 a.m.

79

NOTES

WHEN I HAVE DIED – I chose to write this poem in my husband's voice with the hope of providing comfort and consolation to our children after his death.

AFTER – To Renee, who held my hand and wiped my tears. She lay with me on the bed next to him and talked to George throughout the last coma. She told him she would watch out for me. I am forever grateful.

YOU SHOWED ME – Preparing for George's death well in advance helped me to cope. It was my desire that his death be dignified and have a strong spiritual meaning. We gathered in the mountains after his death for an intimate family ceremony. I set the welcome candle on a table in the middle of the room and lit it one last time. After lighting my taper from it, I extinguished the welcome candle. From my taper, I lit the candle of each family member to represent the continuous cycle of life. I gave everyone a starfish, a symbol of rebirth, and each received a remembrance of George—a photograph from his office, a favorite blanket, a paperweight.

DEAR FATHER – Read at George's funeral Mass, this prayer was written to inspire and comfort our family. During the service, I held on to the drape which covered his coffin, as if holding his hand once again. It was our last goodbye. I prayed for strength to stand, to walk to the pulpit, to speak the words of my heart. My prayers were answered.

MY CAREGIVER FRIEND – This is my wish to each and every caregiver. We *are* joined in spirit and in deed, and it *is* you I pray for every day.

Safe Journey

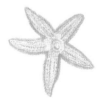

ABOUT THE AUTHOR

Known affectionately as 'j' to her friends, Joyce Marie Sheldon lives in Mooresville, NC, and is the proud mother of one son and six daughters and grandmother to ten grandchildren.

After traveling the journey from fear to faith with her husband George, who died in January 2001, she has made it her mission to nurture the spiritual well-being of others—especially fellow caregivers—through her writing.

She is the creator of CHARACTER ON CALL, a series of character education workshops designed to teach strong decision-making skills to young people. She is also the author of an on-going series of essays entitled "How to Talk to Your Kids About…"

Currently, she is working on her second book, *Love Songs of Man and Mountain*, a collection of tender and romantic prose and poetry.